CHUBBY NO MORE

The Comfort Connection

Build Permanence into Your
Weight Loss Plan in 3 Powerful Steps.

*PROFESSIONAL COPY**

Pamela Aye Simon, MS,RD,LD

*With practice exercises & diagrams of the
CHUBBY NO MORE behavior change model.

authorHOUSE

1663 LIBERTY DRIVE, SUITE 200
BLOOMINGTON, INDIANA 47403
(800) 839-8640
www.authorhouse.com

First published by AuthorHouse 08/13/04

ISBN: 1-4184-2498-6 (e)
ISBN: 1-4184-2499-4 (sc)

Printed in the United States of America
Bloomington, Indiana

This book is printed on acid-free paper.

Cover design in-part by Jenna and Pam Simon

Dedication

These words are dedicated...

To my beautiful daughter and wisest teacher, Jenna, who has an amazing

ability to feel the joy and see the hope in all situations;

To Stanton, who gave me strength;

To my mom, my hero, and a living example of the concepts in this book;

To my dad, who believed I could conquer the impossible;

To my brother, who taught me to challenge everything;

To Dr. Monica, who gave me the chance

to walk above my darkness;

And to all lightworkers everywhere.

Disclaimer

The ideas expressed in this writing are solely those of the author, and do not necessarily represent those of the profession of dietetics as a whole. The concepts presented are based on her professional practice as a registered dietitian and on her personal experience.

The steps and exercises which are explained in this book are not intended to be used as a substitute for medical or psychiatric treatment. In no way should these practices replace care required by physicians or counselors. Prescribed medications should not be changed without direct orders from the prescribing physician.

The book offers guidelines, which may help the reader achieve improved body confidence. These steps do hold the potential of enhancing self esteem, and therefore may contribute to progress made with other self-improvement programs or medical treatment plans.

Forward

With professional expertise and personal knowledge, Pam Aye Simon offers an impressive new vision for lasting weight loss. If you are tired of the endless array of weight loss programs promising results which never seem to last, here is a solid way to ADD POWER to your chosen plan.

The inclusive approach found in CHUBBY NO MORE can complement individual efforts. In fact, all weight loss programs can be strengthened by supplying the often overlooked but crucial keys to successful and permanent results found in this delightful book.

CHUBBY NO MORE should be a companion book for all individuals involved in the weight loss process. Everyone involved could realize greater success and comfort in this process. More importantly, the potential of true, permanent change in weight could finally become reality.

Linda O'Toole, MS,RD

Table of Contents

Introduction.. xiii

Chapter One – The Chubby No More
Power Pieces for Behavior Change 1

Chapter Two
A Salute to the Weight Warriors..7

Chapter Three
I'm Dieting As Fast As I Can.. 11

Chapter Four
All About Me, Me, Me, And You..15

Chapter Five
Buy A New Bathing Suit..19

Chapter Six - Step One
Lose The Guilt 23

Chapter Seven - Step Two
Create New Pay-offs 27

Chapter Eight - Step Three
Paint A New Picture 33

Chapter Nine
Putting It Together 39

Chapter Ten
Q and A..43

Chapter Eleven
Study Guides...53

Chapter Twelve
What I really think… 65

<u>Introduction</u>

When are we going to admit that the weight loss approach used by most diet plans, dieters, and health care professionals SIMPLY IS NOT WORKING? The weight loss process has become distorted and dysfunctional. Individuals may take weight off initially, but those pounds are regained as the months go by. Many times, the well intentioned people who implement various weight loss plans have an ineffective attitude towards the dieter.

The overweight individual is often treated like a naughty child. Guilt, shame and scolding are several of the unhealthy methods used to motivate. The dieter allows this treatment because he or she believes the fault lies within them. The integrity of the dieter is not preserved. Self esteem drops as a result of this treatment, and self confidence for successful weight loss disappears.

The emphasis must change if progress it to be made. Weight loss plans should teach the dieter to trust his or her food behaviors. All blame and scolding must be removed. Instead of striving for "healthy food choices" and "ideal body weight", individuals should be taught how to have a "healthy attitude" towards the food and weight issues. Instead of becoming MORE obsessed with weight and diets, the process of weight control should teach individuals how to think LESS about eating habits &/or weight.

It is possible that the very obsession which runs rampant in society today is making us sicker than any "unhealthy" food choice ever could. Let's stop blaming the food for our eating behaviors.

The lesson to be learned in the process is this: As attention to diet and weight increases, so does the level of difficulty in weight loss maintenance.

The path to permanent weight loss must start with the inside machinery of the individual, i.e. the mind and emotions. Complete and permanent weight control is then possible.

A comparison analogy is this: If your car doesn't start, would you paint and polish the outside of the car to repair the engine? Of course not! Repair must start on the inside.

Success stories are told too soon. Within 2 years of weight loss, ~90% of those individuals who successfully lost weight will gain it back. The weight loss process has become a series of "starter" diets, each restrictive in some way. Success is claimed prematurely. When the individual regains the weight, he or she is often told to go back and re-do what they did, or to try a better weight loss plan, see a psychiatrist, get a support group, etc.

These individuals deserve a better solution. Permanent weight loss results are possible for almost anyone who has made the effort and lost the weight.

In order to reach this goal, the complete solution is this: Build upon the information we already possess. A new and improved diet plan is NOT needed. There are many good weight loss programs on the market. No one weight loss plan can be the answer for everyone. The individual trying to lose weight should choose a weight loss plan with the highest comfort level for him or her.

It is what one does with that chosen plan that determines the outcome.

To reach authentic, lasting weight loss, the process must begin inside the individual. Changes in thoughts and feelings can add the foundational support required if the weight loss is to last.

It is possible to build strength into any weight loss effort. With one simple addition to the chosen diet or plan, a connection can be made to lasting weight loss results.

The power for permanent success is in the three simple steps taught in this book. If practiced along with any weight loss effort, everyone involved in the weight loss process has a chance to experience comfortable, lasting change in weight. In addition, feelings of food deprivation, guilt, frustration and restriction will be replaced by freedom, comfort and self respect.

The change in weight must be integrated into your complete being, as you perceive yourself. If this is not accomplished, you may end up feeling like the analogy written below....

Did I lose weight or am I dressed for a costume party?
You want to lose weight (again), and you are trying the newest of new diets. You tell yourself that THIS TIME you will follow

the diet plan. You try to think positively. This time you will do it. You are excited. .You lose weight with your new efforts, and you feel the battle has been won. Within two years, however, you gain weight. You notice that you have fallen back into your old eating habits. You may have even developed some new bad eating habits! You feel guilty. Your self esteem suffers. You think the failure is your fault.

WRONG!

Weight loss diets do not yield lasting results for this simple reason: your diet isn't a part of the real you. It is someone else's idea. It might work for a year or so; but then it starts to feel like a costume after the costume party is over – really uncomfortable and annoying. Unless you adjust this diet to your likes, cravings, dislikes, forbidden foods, and other personal daily food choice struggles, the new diet will feel like all the others -

IT ISN"T YOU!   THE TRUTH IS : YOUR WEIGHT LOSS
FAILURE IS NOT YOUR FAULT...

You wouldn't expect yourself to keep wearing that costume all
year, would you? Of course not! The same is true of weight loss
diets.

If the eating plan doesn't include your worst (and most loved)
food selections and usual eating behaviors, it probably won't
work over time.

What does work? Getting to the real you and adapting any diet
changes to accommodate your individual style. Let's face it - we
all seem to have times when we eat for the wrong reasons. Your
weight loss diet must provide space for your personal struggles.

It doesn't matter if the diet book or your weight loss professional says something different. If you really want the diet to permanently work this time, you have to...

GET OUT OF THAT SILLY COSTUME!

It Is time to recover from the damaging effects of dysfunctional diets.

When your diet becomes part of the REAL YOU, success comes more easily, and feelings of comfort and confidence prevail. I am here to help you finally feel the comfort you deserve.

Pam Aye Simon

Imagine yourself light enough
to fly up to the stars.
If this challenges you
let us surround you with comfort.
When your comfort is deep enough
you will find the wings to fly.
-pas

Chapter One – The Chubby No More Power Pieces for Behavior Change

Weight loss results rarely last more than 2 years. *Why?*

There have been vital pieces missing from the weight loss process. The existing methods for implementing weight loss plans leave out the most important steps.

These missing parts have the potential of being "power pieces" for behavior change. The addition of these missing pieces to weight loss efforts is a key component in the conversion of temporary weight loss results to permanent change.

Eating behavior and weight loss results are affected deeply by mental & emotional blocks to behavior change.

With the simple method found in this book, these blocks can be easily removed. In fact, with practice, the blocks can be transformed into power pieces.

The powerful effects of these mental/emotional issues are not addressed in most weight loss plans. When these vital parts are added, the possibility of lasting weight loss dramatically increases.

Resolution of mental & emotional blocks is key to permanent results. The following three steps form the foundation of the Chubby No More Behavior Change Model. The diagrams illustrate the ineffective behavior change model used by most weight loss plans, and the permanent effects of the Chubby No More model.

1) GUILT – GET RID OF IT

Guilt feelings about food & weight are not helpful at all. In the long run, these feelings will lower the success potential of the individual.

For permanent results, all food guilt must be cleared away. Guilt feelings can damage self esteem so much that the individual unconsciously gives up the effort to lose weight.

2) **FAILURE PAYOFFS – CREATE SUCCESS PAYOFFS**

There are rewards that result from being overweight. Feelings of comfort and safety with an overweight body can unconscientiously keep the individual stuck.

Unless this comfort is changed, the individual will continually regress to the old weight. The same good feelings must be created for the same individual in a thinner body.

Pamela Aye Simon, MS,RD,LD

3) NEGATIVE BODY IMAGE – CHANGE TO POSITIVE

A positive outcome should be expected. Imagination and visualization are tools for success in this step.

This is not as easy as it sounds. It involves a skill that must be practiced daily. Most of us are trained to be realistic, to not get hopes up, to stay grounded, etc. Forget that! The habit of picturing oneself with a successful outcome is vital to making weight loss permanent.

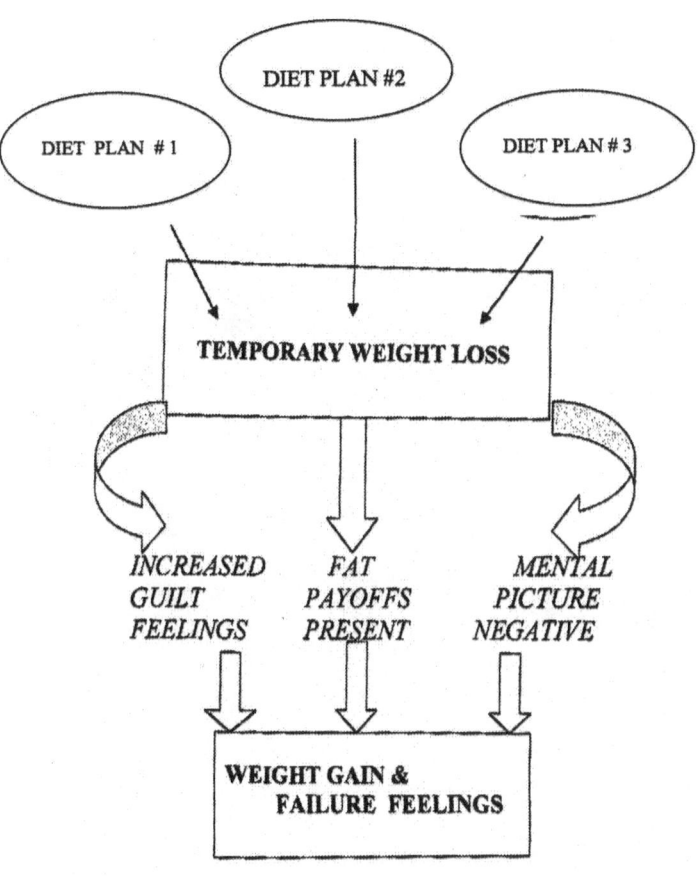

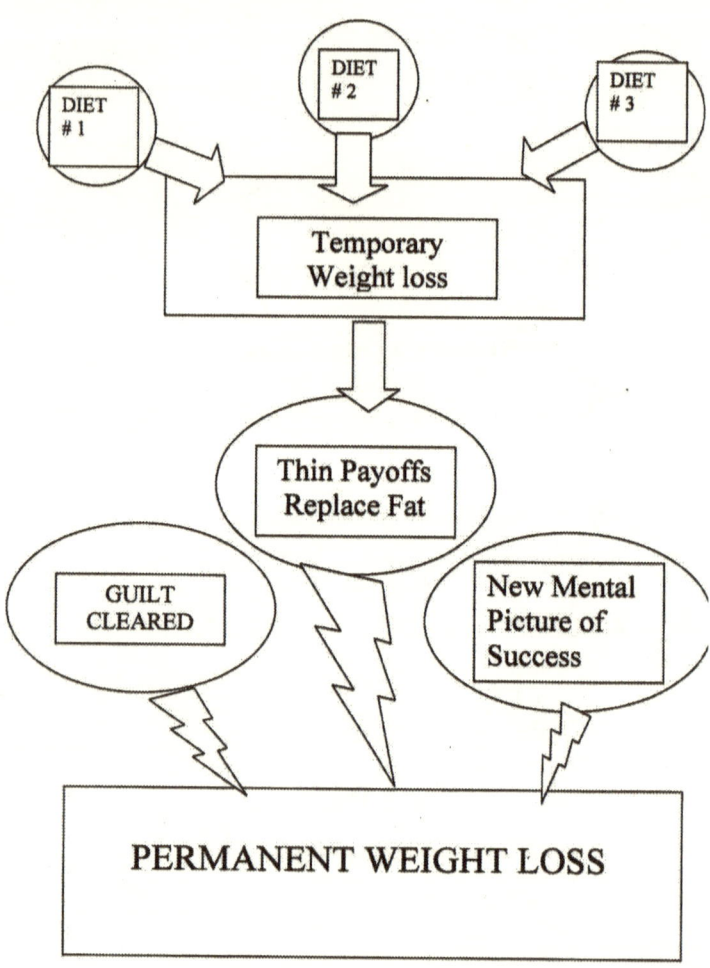

DIET #1

DIET #2

DIET #3

Temporary Weight loss

Thin Payoffs Replace Fat

GUILT CLEARED

New Mental Picture of Success

PERMANENT WEIGHT LOSS

Chapter Two
A Salute to the Weight Warriors

How do you feel about your body image right now? Do you carry around negative feelings about your weight, your fitness level, or your eating habits?

If you have moments in your day when you feel guilty about what you eat, what you weigh, or how you look, this book is for you. If you are too tired to try another exercise class, read on. Even if you refuse to alter your eating plan, or feel like you just found the perfect diet, there is something here for you.

But first, a tribute is in order, and is long overdue.

For all of you who have struggled with weight loss plans,

I salute you and your fighting spirit.

You are remarkable.

And yet....

You are rarely given credit for the battles you fight. More often

than not, you are blamed for not fighting hard enough.

You seem to bounce back.

If one weight loss method doesn't work, you don't give up.

You get the strength to try another.

Your self- esteem suffers terribly, yet much of your pain is kept

hidden. You don't blame others for the struggle.

You tend to place all the blame on yourself.

You may have years of great success and the highest hope that

the battle has been won. But just when you think you can relax,

the weight battle begins again.

This book is a salute to you. You are the embodiment of the spirits of hope, persistence and courage.

You are a hero.

In this book, I offer you a different path - one that soothes and comforts you.

This path provides a connection between you

and the body image of your dreams.

The element that has been missing from your efforts is the very

thing you thought you couldn't have –

increased feelings of deep comfort - to replace the pain and

guilt.

Enough with the guilt.

Enough with the pain.

Right now, you need comfort.

Then you can get down to the business of weight loss.

Chapter Three
I'm Dieting As Fast As I Can

Losing weight can be a challenge for just about anyone. Maintaining weight loss for more than two years seems to baffle the best of us (dieters and health professionals alike).

The failure rate of maintaining weight loss is not anyone's fault. The individuals who are trying to lose the weight commonly blame the failure on themselves. In fact, the overweight individual is indeed blamed by well-intentioned family members, friends, and health care professionals.

We need a much more healing approach. We need to build, not blame. The fault lies not with the individual, the program nor the professional.

***In fact, the inability to achieve and/or maintain weight loss has
very little to do with what you eat.***

In the pages of this book, the reader will learn how to strengthen
weight loss efforts in five to ten minutes a day of delightful mental
exercises.

That is what it did for me.

This is my story. I survived the struggle, and I lived the solution.
I have endured more weight loss diets, pills and exercise routines
than I can remember. I have survived addictive and strange eating
behaviors and consuming preoccupation with my weight... but
not anymore.

I am also a registered dietitian with years of experience in the
weight loss counseling field. Today, when one of my clients says:
"Give me a diet, I have to lose weight," I refuse. I cannot add any

more guilt to the shoulders of someone who may still be blaming himself/herself for the failure of past diets.

The diet by itself just won't work. Pounds might come off, but they may as easily come back. Within 2 years, the weight will be regained and feelings of failure and guilt will increase.

This failure isn't the fault of the individual or of the weight loss program. Something has been missing.

For all of the suffering, hard work and progress – including various diet plans, fitness programs, surgical procedures and diet pills, weight change just doesn't seem to last.

We have all tried to find the reason, but it has been a challenge to see the big picture. As a result, most of our programs address the physical change desired, but we have not addressed the vital process of mental and emotional adjustment to the change.

Mental and emotional readiness for weight change is so important, it very well could be the key to unlocking long-term, successful weight loss. There should be as much emphasis on changing the inside of the individual so that he or she can prepare for, and become comfortable with, the good body changes.

It is really the whole person who needs attention – the body, the mind and the spirit.

Chapter Four
All About Me, Me, Me, And You

A very crucial part of the process has been missing. In the world of weight loss programs, the addition of this part could change the long-term results completely.

I found this answer by living through the problem. .It took many years, but today I am able to live without thoughts of food and body weight, and with no feelings of guilt.

My first dieting experience was "The Grapefruit and Cottage Cheese Diet." (I went on this one with my dad.) The last was the "Eat a Box of Cookies-a-Day Diet." (This one was my very own invention – but it worked as well as any other.) There were many other weight loss diets in between. The "Eat only Peas Diet," and the "Ten Snacks-a-Day (but no meals) Diet" were two of the most memorable.

Then there were all the exercise plans, like the "Yoga Stretch (between meals of lettuce) program," and the "Run-Around-the-Yard Plan" (my mom's idea).

And guess what? I did lose weight...

...again, and again, and again.

And I gained back the lost weight...

...again, and again, and again.

I had to face the reality that my approach to weight loss wasn't working. Sure, I could lose weight. But I kept finding it again - along with lots of guilt. I kept doing the same thing over and over and expecting different results.

This miserable cycle of ... diet>>>>>weight-loss>>>>>>

whoops!>>>>>weight-gain>>>>diet ... was ... what? ... not working?

After many exhausting years of dieting and exercise activities, I knew I was missing something. There was something missing from my various weight loss efforts. There will always be another eating plan, pill, or exercise program which promises to be more successful for weight loss than all the others. There will always be one that looks different, one that promises to hold the secret.

Finally, I said to myself: " ***No More.*** "

I was damaged by my failed diet attempts. I was disappointed by temporary results. I wanted to stop this craziness. I felt like a jilted lover. The relationship I had with my body image and food was highly dysfunctional.

I was losing my self worth...... one calorie at a time. I wanted to live life. I was weary of driving down the street and noticing the advertisements for food and restaurants...instead of looking up at the trees and sky.

I was tired of counting calories.

I longed to count the stars instead...

I longed for a bigger life....

Chapter Five
Buy A New Bathing Suit

Readiness. I hadn't prepared the mental and emotional me for the physical changes. Becoming a thinner person wasn't totally comfortable for me because I wasn't used to it. My internal body mold was too big now for the thinner, physical me.

When I did lose weight, somewhere inside me I FELT STRANGE.

I felt like I lost weight but forgot to buy a new bathing suit! I felt a draft! I felt exposed!

There was too much space. There was a space inside me that needed to be filled. I felt mentally/emotionally overweight even though I was physically thinner.

Although I loved being the thinner person, there was a part of me that wanted to bring back the *overweight-me*. Deep down, I felt safer when my body size stayed the same. The *overweight-me* was someone I had known a long time. Of course I wanted to be thinner!

I just wasn't sure I wanted to hang out with the new *thinner-body-me*. This *thinner-body-me* was a stranger. Sure, I was now living in her body. But I didn't feel as safe as before. She was unfamiliar and threatening.

I wasn't sure I was prepared for what this thinner person would make me do. What if she signed me up for power yoga, or made me give up chocolate, or wanted to "dress for success" everyday.....or worse? ***Was I ready for all this?*** Attaining permanent weight loss requires the development of deep comfort feelings and thoughts about being a thinner person.

The major reason for weight-loss failure over time has everything to do with an individual's state of readiness for living in a thinner body. On some level, I still saw myself as the out-of-shape me, the person who believed it when someone told her that she would "get fat just like Daddy."

Over the years, I got a lot of practice with this feeling. It was safe and familiar. I was used to it… like a worn sweat suit, or an old shoe. And unless I could change my emotional comfort level to include a better-body me, weight loss wouldn't feel OK..

Just as in any construction project, the foundation MUST be in place for the rest of the building to remain stable. A permanent weight change requires foundational work as well. *The weight loss process does not automatically include a plan for emotional adjustment – you have to take care of this.*

Just because you may have wanted to be thinner for a long time, don't assume you will naturally feel wonderful when it happens. FEELING COMFORTABLE with the changes that come with weight loss success is not automatic - it takes practice.

In the chapters that follow, you will learn how to add this crucial (but simple) method to your existing lifestyle with only 5-10 minutes a day of delightful mental exercises.

This method teaches how to become emotionally and mentally ready for success in weight management. Finally, you can stop attracting the weight we have lost. Changes in the body require changes in thinking and feeling habits if they are to last.

Chapter Six - Step One
Lose The Guilt

Weight loss plans and guilt feelings are supposed to go together –

right? And these guilt feelings are really good motivators, right?

NO. In fact, the exact opposite is true. You cannot live in guilt

and have lasting successful weight loss at the same time. In order

to lay the foundation for that success you have to see and feel

yourself as a very strong, courageous and amazing person. Guilt

doesn't serve a purpose. STOP FEELING GUILTY about weight

and eating habits.

The first step in the process of growing comfortable with success is

this: shake off the guilt. You have control over this. Guilt feelings

are just a habit, and as silly as it sounds, you have to practice

living without them.

Guilt takes many forms. For example, guilt tells you to dwell on what you should have done, or didn't do in situations regarding eating or exercise (like, "I shouldn't have eaten...." Or "I should be going to the health club...") STOP. You do not deserve to be beaten up by guilt. It serves no purpose.

Many individuals think they must feel guilty for unrestricted eating behaviors so that they do not lose control completely. That doesn't happen. In fact, with the guilt gone, more confidence gives a greater sense of control over eating habits and weight.

Losing the guilt can help you to feel better about yourself in many ways. This will increase your comfort level with success. Guilt about eating and weight only serves to add pounds in the long run. Sure, at first, guilt and fear may help to get you started. But, in the long run, it hinders positive results, and may do more to rob you of weight loss success than almost any other influence.

You have to get rid of guilt, and still feel comfortable.

But how do you get rid of guilt in a simple way?

It just takes practice.

The exercise that is most helpful is described below. Remember that you are undoing years of habitual guilt feelings. To stop the guilt habit you need two things: repetition and written words. This combination has a powerful effect.

Practice for 2 minutes each day, with the following exercise: With paper and pen,

write the words "Right now, I feel free from all guilt about my eating behavior. I feel a sense of comfort and trust instead of guilt.," (You can get specific with this.) Practice this exercise for 1 minute each morning and 1 minute each evening.

This may feel silly at first. In time, however, what you write will eventually reach your feelings. You will actually feel energized as guilt drops away. You are now clearing the way for the next step.

<u>EXERCISES</u>

1) List 5 foods that you feel guilty or frustrated about eating, wanting to eat, sneaking to eat, eating too much of, etc.

2) Write a statement about your feelings that contradict the guilt (even if you don't feel this at first), such as : "I enjoyed that food, I'm happy I let myself eat that food, I feel free to eat any food" and so on.

Chapter Seven - Step Two
Create New Pay-offs

There are times when everyone feels like a scared child. This is the piece of us that wants to stay in the same, safe place .It is a quiet voice in our hearts that seeks to protect us from emotional annihilation. For some of us, the voice is too soft to hear. Others are well aware of its sound. Either way, its influence seems to be quite powerful.

For example, there are some aspects to being over weight that may help increase feelings of safety and comfort. Recognizing this fact and changing it has been crucial in helping me and others connect to permanent weight loss. Think about it - you have probably lived with your overweight-self for a while. It is familiar and it seems safe. And, believe it or not, there are some positive pay-offs for remaining this way. One obvious pay-off is that you can keep things the same, which offers a certain level of comfort. You don't have to change your activities, eating habits, or exercise routine... the list goes on.

These pay-offs are hard to give up, because they comfort you and protect you from the unknown. Some aren't even quite on the conscious level. And guess what - we all have these! This brings us to the next step.

You need to identify some of these pay-offs. You do not need to analyze deeply or take very long to do this. You don't need to come up with all of the details. These comfort areas exist, and should be recognized. What makes you want to stay in the overweight zone?

Here are some examples of pay-offs you may identify:

-You don't have to worry about being in style

-You have a reason to stay in the house

-You don't have to go swimming with …

And so on. Do this once

Then move on to the second part of this step. This part is very important. Imagine that you are the thin person you long to be. What are some of the wonderful ways you will feel the benefits of being thinner?

These benefits need to become real for you. You need to create new, comfortable and soothing pay-offs for the thinner person you are becoming. Again, this takes practice. Feelings of comfort are key.

If you haven't spent much time in your life as a thin person, practice this step diligently. You are helping that little scared kid inside you feel more secure with changes that occur in your body weight.

You have to picture some rewards you may experience as a thinner person that are comforting, soothing and wonderful - new comfort pay-offs.

Some examples would be:

-I hear my daughter whisper in my ear that I look beautiful

-I have more energy when I wake up in the morning

-I try on jeans that are 2 sizes smaller, and they fit!

Now for the exercise which puts this step into action:

Write this down with pen and paper:

Imagine some of the rewards you might experience when you have a better body. Are some of these new pay-offs scary or threatening? Cross these out. Are some of the pay-offs really comforting to think about? Write these down again. Be totally aware of how you feel when you imagine the pay-offs.

Do this for 1 minute each morning and one minute in the evening. You need to be able to come up with at least five better-body pay-offs that feel really good. Keep doing this daily.

<u>EXERCISES</u>

1) List 3 chubby-you pay-offs which make you feel comfortable.

2) List 3 thinner-you pay-offs you want really badly

Chapter Eight - Step Three
Paint A New Picture

This is a great step. It takes the old phrase: "you are what you eat," and expands it to the more meaningful and delightful words: "you are what you think (feel, believe, etc)." The successful outcome of your weight loss plan depends mainly upon the way you think about yourself.

If you have lots of negative images of yourself and your weight, these images need to be changed. They are old pictures, and need to be replaced with new ones. You need to become emotionally comfortable with your mental pictures of the new you. The great news is this: With practice, these new images can become part of you, and will then affect how you respond to your desire to change.

The more you practice thinking of yourself as a beautiful example of success, the better chance you have of losing weight and keeping it off- and with a lot more comfort.

Please practice this step for 2 minutes in the morning and two minutes in the evening.

With pen and paper, record the following:

Imagine that you are the thinner person you desire to be. Describe yourself in positive ways as if it were happening in the present, like "I am thin and confident...". Imagine what you are wearing, doing, saying, feeling, thinking, etc. Imagine in color.

Your feelings are especially important, as are all the details you can picture. This may seem ridiculous at first. Don't let that stop you. Your mental picture of the physical person you want to be may feel unrealistic, but shouldn't seem impossible. It may feel slightly foreign, but shouldn't create stress. With practice, the best image for you will become clear.

Do not give up on the practice of this step for anything. You may have days, hours, moments when it seems like nonsense. Practice anyway. The negativity will pass. You may not have the time to put anything in writing. If that is the case, close your eyes and think this step. Do this step each day, no matter what.

Continue to hold the image of who you want to be in your mind's eye. As you spend time daily with this mental picture, you will feel much more comfortable with the new you.

Never give this up.

Weight loss success will naturally follow. Other great changes may happen. You may experience much greater ease in following your chosen weight loss plan, fitness program, etc. You may want to take a break from defined eating plans. You may even find you have an inherent desire to make healthier choices.

Why?

Your new emotional comfort level is now connecting you to the dreams you once thought impossible. And this is only the beginning...

EXERCISE

Close your eyes. Imagine yourself 5 pounds thinner. Imagine a place at home or work doing a task you enjoy. Imagine what you're wearing, who you are talking to, etc.

Chapter Nine
Putting It Together

Finally, let's put all the steps together:

1. LOSE THE GUILT

Practice for 2 minutes each day:

Write the words "I am free of guilt about my weight/eating/exercise habits today," (or you your own wording for the same message) for 1 minute each morning and 1 minute each evening. The words you write will eventually reach your feelings.

2. CREATE NEW PAY-OFFS

Practice for 2 minutes twice a day:

Write *some of the rewards you might experience when you have a better body. Are some of these new pay-offs scary or threatening? Cross these out. Are some of the pay-offs really comforting to think about? Write these down again. Be totally aware of how you feel when you imagine the pay-offs. You need to be able to come up with at least five better-body pay-offs that feel really good.*

3. PAINT A BETTER PICTURE

Practice this step for 2 minutes twice a day:

Record the following: imagine that you are the thinner person you desire to be.

Describe yourself in detailed, positive ways, as if it were happening in the present (like "I am at a party at my house, wearing a black dress, and feeling thin and confident...". Imagine what you are wearing, doing, saying, feeling, thinking, etc. Imagine in color.

Your feelings are especially important, as are all the details you

can picture. Come up with as many different scenarios as you can.

With practice, the best image for you will become clear.

In conclusion: your thoughts and written words are yours. Keep them away from the eyes and ears of anyone who may not understand. Don't allow any outside opinions to minimize or criticize your work.

You may not always be able to practice the steps in a quiet place with a pen and paper. That doesn't matter. Take mental quiet time and do the exercises in your imagination. Your goal is to become familiar and comfortable with an image of yourself as successful in permanent weight loss. You may use variations of the above steps, or add strategies of your own creation.

Finally, the process of developing the comfort connection with successful weight loss is simple, but not easy. Daily practice, repetition, and your own written words give power to your efforts, and bring success closer to you.

Chapter Ten
Q and A

Q.

Do I have to practice this method for the rest of my life for lasting results?

A.

Yes and no. With daily practice, the positive body image you have created will take hold on a deeper level. The process becomes part of who you are. Over time, the positive images automatically replace negative ones.

But no matter what, you need to do the exercises everyday, even when things are going great, and especially after you have lost the desired amount of weight.

Q.

How long do I have to practice before the positive images become automatic?

A.

That depends on how severe your negative body imagery has become. On average, at the end of 3 months of daily practice, the process should be integrated into your thoughts. It should seem easier to do.

Q.

What should my eating plan be while I am learning all of this?

A.

You can follow any healthy food plan of your choice. But you need to relax about eating, and to not feel guilty about your eating during this time.

Q.

What if I feel just too silly imagining myself as thin?

A.

Take baby steps. The first week, imagine yourself 3 pounds thinner, then 5, 7, and so on. It will work. If you are not ready yet, acknowledge and respect that feeling inside yourself. You will know when the time is right.

Q.

Why do some people have a lot less trouble staying thin than other people?

A.

No one knows the total answer to that question. It may be a combination of factors, like genetics, eating habits, metabolic rate, etc.

For most of us, however, I believe we can still change our weight loss success by working with body image.

In my family, my grandmother, great grandmother, and great grandfather were very overweight, as was my Dad. If I can fight a pattern like this, so can you.

Q.

Can't you just tell me specifically how many calories I need to lose weight, and then plan meals for me? Isn't that what a dietitian does? I just need you to tell me what to do.

A.

I do not provide this service for a very good reason. IT DOESN'T WORK! The more restrictive we become, the less likely we are to attain weight loss that lasts more than 2 years. There are many less restrictive diets available. If you need a structured food plan, make sure you choose one that is the most comfortable for you. But, along with any food plan, using the three step method in this book can help ease the pain of the process . From my experience, the diet and method used together could greatly enhance your chances of achieving and maintaining weight loss.

Q.

What about the supplements that claim to burn fat or carbohydrates? Couldn't that help also?

A.

If there were a pill which offered a safe and permanent solution to weight loss, we would ALL be taking it, wouldn't we? I sure would! As a professional registered dietitian, I can't recommend these products for my clients, simply because research evidence on efficacy and effectiveness is not yet complete. It is possible that any number of products have potential in the weight loss area.

Q.

Is it OK to just accept myself as a heavy person, and stop trying to be the thin person I am not?

A.

What a great question! Yes. It is time for all of us to accept ourselves for what we are today. I should have put that factor in the chapter on losing the guilt. The great thing about accepting the present you, is that once you do this, you can feel and see more clearly whether you actually WANT to lose weight. You are allowed to decide NOT to try to lose weight now.

Q.

You say in the book to ease up on eating restrictions. I am a binger. If I ease up, there is no telling how much I will eat. It is scary.

A.

If the eating really scares you, the first action to be taken is to consult with an eating disorder specialist. A true eating disorder can be dangerous, and may have brain chemistry abnormalities. There are some great medications that can provide substantial help once an eating disorder diagnosis is made.

Otherwise, it seems that most people who have been restricting food intake do experience feelings of anger at being deprived of the amounts of favorite foods desired.

These feelings can build frustration levels to the point where eating control gives way to saying "the hell with this," followed by binging behavior.

There actually is a solution to this kind of binging. This solution may sound like the exact opposite of what you think you should do, but it worked for me… really worked. And it WAS SCARY!

Here it is: for the next 2 weeks, have no restrictions on your eating. Eat anything you want, at any time you want, in any quantity you wish. You won't believe what happens next. You will actually grow tired of the foods you have been longing for, and you will have no feelings of deprivation. It will feel comfortable.

You also will have no reason to binge anymore. And please do not force yourself to eat 3 meals a day during this time, or have all the basic food groups at a meal, or whatever else you might try to do. You will have time for all of that healthy stuff after this problem is addressed. Do, however, take a daily multivitamin with minerals.

Q.

The method taught in this book seems like it might work to help me in other areas of my life. Is this possible ?

A.

Absolutely! I actually developed this method in order to help me perform music in front of audiences with more joy and composure. I had such great success, that I literally apply the techniques to all of my challenges. You can do this also – just change the wording and mental pictures as needed.

PRETEND

It had been such a long day...

with kids and pets to care for

and messes to clean up...

I almost missed it...

I didn't really expect an answer

when I casually asked my young child,

What is the meaning of the word... PRETEND?"

One word is all she said...

BELIEVE

Chapter Eleven
Study Guides

STEP ONE:

Describe five things about which you have been feeling guilty regarding your eating, fitness or weight. After each description, write a phrase which will help you lose this guilt. (For example, "I will not criticize myself for eating cookies today.")

GUILT #1

COMFORT STATEMENT

GUILT #2

COMFORT STATEMENT

GUILT #3

COMFORT STATEMENT

GUILT #4

COMFORT STATEMENT

GUILT #5

COMFORT STATEMENT

STEP TWO

List three comfort pay-offs for the over-weight you, and how you
can picture living without each:

PAY-OFF #1 - CHUBBY

PAY-OFF #2 - CHUBBY

PAY-OFF #3 - CHUBBY

STEP TWO continued

List and describe in detail five soothing pay-offs for the new, thinner you:

PAY-OFF #1 - THIN

PAY-OFF #2 - THIN

PAY-OFF #3 - THIN

PAY-OFF #4 - THIN

PAY-OFF #5 - THIN

STEP THREE:

Imagine five scenarios with you as a thinner person.

Take your time with this one. Close your eyes if possible. Let your imagination soar! Describe every detail of each situation.

Picture yourself actually inside the situations, as a person who feels fit and confident, a person who is an example of permanent weight loss. Who are you with? Where are you (describe the setting)? What are you thinking? What are you feeling? What are you wearing? Make these situations similar to those you encounter now, but imagine that you are thinner in these pictures.

SCENARIO #1

Setting:

Clothes:

Who is present:

Conversation

Your feelings:

<u>SCENARIO #2</u>

Setting:

Clothes:

Who you are with:

Conversation:

Your feelings:

SCENARIO #3

Setting:

Clothes:

Who is present:

Conversation

Your feelings"

<u>SCENARIO #4</u>

Setting:

Clothes:

Who is present:

Conversation:

Your feelings

<u>SCENARIO #5</u>

Setting:

Clothes:

Who is present:

Conversation:

Your feelings

Chapter Twelve
What I really think...

I am a rebel dietitian. I used to be a traditional professional, who gave conventional advice for weight loss. ..but I never saw a client who achieved permanent, life-long weight loss results. It is time for all of us to admit that the present approach doesn't work.

I hold many unconventional beliefs. Below, I have listed a few statements which represent these beliefs. Before I make these statements, however, I must say that I respect and admire all the hard-working people who have helped countless individuals with weight loss problems, and I truly am grateful for The American Dietetic Association for its continuing efforts to educate the public in healthier eating habits. I am also extremely grateful to everyone at Rush University for giving me the confidence to question traditional teachings.

Now…for a few challenging thoughts…

>Let's be realistic. It is no longer probable that families will have quality time" together at a meal! Get away from the food table for quality time. Eating dysfunction in parents is played out at the table - and our kids are suffering.

>Following the "Food Guide Pyramid" for a balanced diet reminds me of college in a way. Anyone out there remember Sorority Hell Week?

>Throw out that scale. It has become an object of evil.

> Eat your favorite foods proudly, and savor every bite. After months or years of diet torture, you deserve to enjoy your favorite foods!

> If someone tells you to keep a "food journal," just say no.

>The first rule of thumb for permanent weight loss is to NEVER, EVER WEIGH YOURSELF. The more often you weigh yourself, the less often you seem to achieve weight loss. No one knows why, but why take the chance?

> The second rule of thumb is to NEVER write down the foods you eat daily. Charting what you eat daily seems to increase the amount of food you eat daily. This is also a mystery.

> Moderation is just a fantasy. There is really no such thing.

>One of the characteristics of insanity is to do the same thing over and over and expect different results. To lose weight, many of us diet over and over and expect different results. Hmmm......there's a message here...

>If you want to watch me eat a whole package of Oreos in a short period of time please do the following: Tell me that I must stop eating Oreo Cookies. Then sit back and enjoy the show.

> If you want to watch me eat Oreo cookies in moderation, please do the following: Tell me that I can eat any amount of Oreos at anytime. That wrecks the fun totally

> I'm confused. Experts say that we should have a 30% fat diet (or less) from vegetable sources. Twinkies are only 30% fat, all from vegetable sources. What's the problem?

> The Ideal Body Weight Tables were originally the guess-work of an insurance company. DO NOT take them seriously.

> You are not the food police for your family. Stop talking about healthy food choices, junk food, weight control, etc. And most

of all, DO NOT try to control what your kids (or other family members) eat. If food becomes an issue in your family, you just might be a setting the stage for an eating disorder.

>It is time to tell everyone else in your life to lay off about your eating world. No one has a right to criticize, or to offer comments, advice, etc. This is your private space - OFF LIMITS. No one, including yourself, is allowed to beat you up with criticisms in this area. Demand integrity.

>There is no such thing as junk food or fast food. There is just food. We need to stop with the labels.

>Here's a challenge for you – try to have normal conversations and interactions with the usual people in your life, but, for 2 weeks, try to make absolutely NO reference to diet (any kind), food, recipes, weight, - get it? Just try to have meaningful conversations

without food as a topic. Also, do not listen to or read about diets and weight for those 2 weeks. Impossible?

> We treat ourselves as adults in many areas of our lives – finance, job responsibilities, marriage, parenting, etc. Why, then do we treat ourselves like children in the eating/weight area – with self-scolding, deprivation, punishment through exercise, and so on. We all need to reclaim our integrity. Only then can we make real progress.

Every individual, regardless of weight or eating habits, deserves to know the following basic freedoms: the freedom to eat and enjoy food again; the freedom to never feel guilty for doing so…the freedom to say 'no' to diets; the freedom to say 'yes' to oneself.

About The Author

Pamela Aye Simon is a registered, licensed dietitian in private practice in Illinois. She received her Bachelor of Science Degree from Indiana University of Pennsylvania, and earned her Master of Science Degree in Clinical Nutrition from Rush University in Chicago, Illinois. Since then, Ms. Aye Simon has been active in the area of nutrition research and weight control.

From her positions as a research dietitian implementing dietary counseling for clinical trials, to study manager in charge of monitoring the operations of a feeding study, her experiences have allowed her a unique prospective on the weight loss dilemma.

In addition, her private practice and her own personal journey through the world of programs for weight control make this author an excellent resource for others who struggle or work with the weight loss process.

Ms. Aye Simon has co-authored numerous research articles, which have been published in scientific journals.

Contact information:

Pam welcomes comments and questions. For all

communications, including seminar and lecture requests, please

contact her via

e-mail at:

psimon36@aol.com

or visit

www.chubbynomore.org

MOMMY HELP

There was a day, not long ago..

I felt alone and scared.

I needed help with everything,

but help just wasn't there.

A mom I was, and had to be.

I needed to be strong.

"Please help!" I prayed.

And then I heard…

"He's been here all along."

I listened to my child's voice,

and was surprised to hear…

the wisdom of the ages

whispering in my ear.

I stared into my child's eyes

and was amazed to see..

the love and strength of Heaven

waiting there for me.

Remembering that life is more

than healthy food and weight…

I stop and feel the moment,

before it is too late.

(PAS)

www.ingramcontent.com/pod-product-compliance
Lightning Source LLC
Chambersburg PA
CBHW030404290526
45785CB00004B/1893